love

Josanne

X

Brave Heart

JOANNE GILLESPIE

CENTURY
London   Sydney   Auckland   Johannesburg

First published in 1989 by Century Hutchinson Ltd,
Brookmount House, 62–65 Chandos Place,
Covent Garden, London WC2N 4NW

Century Hutchinson Australia Pty Ltd,
89–91 Albion Street, Surry Hills, Sydney,
New South Wales 2010, Australia

Century Hutchinson New Zealand Limited,
PO Box 40-086, Glenfield, Auckland 10, New Zealand

Century Hutchinson South Africa (Pty) Ltd,
PO Box 337, Bergvlei, 2012 South Africa

British Library Cataloguing in Publication Data
Gillespie, Joanne
    Brave Heart: the diary of a nine-year-old girl
    who refused to die
    1. Man. Serious illnesses. Personal adjustment. Biography.
    I. Title
    155.9'16'0924
    ISBN 0-7126-3461-4

All illustrations used in this book are by Joanne Gillespie,
except for the Brave Heart Lion illustration on p. 8,
and the hospital illustration on the back cover and p. 33
which are by Sarah Gillespie.

Care Bears are the trademark of
Those Characters From Cleveland Inc

Designed by Clare Clements and edited by Annie Norton
Typeset in Palatino by DP Photosetting, Aylesbury, Bucks
Printed and bound in Italy by OFSA Spa, Milan

FOREWORD

It seems to me that whenever there is a lull in the few social gatherings which I am asked to attend, someone is bound to turn to me and ask brightly, 'And who was your favourite guest on *Wogan*?' I stand there, mumchance. I can scarcely remember who I talked to last Monday, much less carry around a Top Ten Guest List in my head. When you've done over 600 shows and talked to over 2,000 guests in four years, faces tend to get a bit blurred.

I hope that I'll never become blasé about talking with the great and the good; the leaders of men, temporal and spiritual; the legendary stars of Hollywood and the Haunted Fish Tank. To meet the celluloid heroes and heart-throbs of my youth is a never-to-be-forgotten experience: June Allyson, Bette Davis, Jane Russell, James Stewart, Kirk Douglas, Charlton Heston... A privilege to share a stage with Stevie Wonder, Paul McCartney, Jessye Norman, Kiri Te Kanawa, Luciano Pavarotti, Placido Domingo...

Yet, amid all the glitter and glamour, the guests that remain in my memory are the 'ordinary' people – the ones whose courage, bravery and grace under pressure make them very far from 'ordinary'. The youngest of these, and therefore the most remarkable, for her spirit, resilience and sheer willpower, was a young lady I met late in 1988, Joanne Gillespie. This is her book. Read it, weep, and exult that such a spirit lives. Brave Heart, indeed!

Terry Wogan

ACKNOWLEDGEMENTS

I want to say a big thank you to everyone who has helped me – all the doctors and nurses in Middlesbrough General Hospital, especially Mr Nath my surgeon, my family and all my friends. And a very special thank you to my lovely sister, Sarah, because she has been very good and helped me a lot.

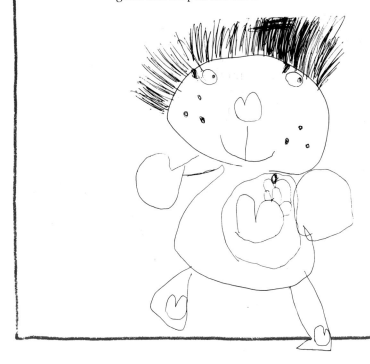

'Brave Heart Lion' by Sarah Gillespie

INTRODUCTION

by Joanne's Mother

Joanne was a very good baby, and a healthy child. We could never have guessed that anything like this was going to hit us. She was our first child, and was born in North Tees Hospital on December 5th, 1977. But at her birth we both thought something had gone wrong. I'd had a caesarean, and Peter was waiting in a little side room. I remember seeing him an hour-and-a-half after the birth and saying 'Is it a boy or a girl?' And Peter didn't know. That worried us – but it was simply that the shifts had changed just after Joanne was born and so nobody had thought to tell Peter!

She has Peter's temperament, his sense of humour, she's not afraid to talk to new people. As a baby she always hated going to bed. We had some friends who would come round once a week when she was tiny, and she'd be up until 11 pm. She wanted to be where we were. So she'd be sitting up in her bed all evening.

From very early days she was very musical. Neither of us is especially musical, though we like music. But she's got a real sense of rhythm. On holiday, she's the first on the dance floor. She can move to whatever the tune – foxtrot, waltz, jive – she doesn't need a partner. She's a dancer, and it's kept her going through her illness. The girls' interest in ballet has given

BRAVE HEART

us an interest too – neither of us had been to the ballet before.

Sarah was born four years after Joanne, on July 15th, 1981. It was another caesarean, but it was much nicer because Peter could hold her straight afterwards, even before she'd been cleaned up. I don't remember any time when Joanne was jealous of her little sister. She'd always liked babies and was a proper little mother. She used to help talcum powder Sarah, and she'd try to push the pram, though she couldn't reach it. We used to go out with me pushing Sarah in the pram, and Joanne pushing one of her dolls in its pram.

The girls may fight with each other now, but Joanne won't let anyone go after Sarah. Sarah's the same; she feels she's got a responsibility for Joanne since she's been ill, and she'll try to protect her. Since the operations some children at school haven't been kind to Joanne. There was one little boy who was taunting her, calling her 'baldy', but she saw the Head come up and stand behind him and she just waited until he stopped and the Head gave him a telling off! Joanne doesn't want me to interfere – she wants to be treated the same as all the other children. The teachers gave her a special chair to sit on at assembly but she wouldn't sit on it – she wanted to sit on the floor just like all the others.

When she first started having the headaches I thought nothing of it, though my mother and I do suffer from migraines. We'd never had any worries about her health, though she had had her tonsils taken out, and she'd had a totally benign fatty lump removed from her side. But the headaches got worse and worse, and our GP tried everything. GPs aren't specialists, and they might not see many brain tumours in their whole career, so he tried everything else first.

Then she started being sick every time we went out in the car. Our GP prescribed some medicine and warned us that it had side effects. So the day

BRAVE HEART

– I remember it was a Friday – that she became paralysed down her side, Peter worried at first that he might just have given her the wrong dose of medicine by mistake. We didn't have an appointment so we had to wait until the end of the surgery to be seen, but as soon as he saw Joanne the GP told us to go staight to North Tees Hospital and not to wait for an ambulance.

By the time we got there Joanne was beginning to feel better, the paralysis was going and she started laughing and joking just like she always does. Peter was worrying that they'd send her home because they couldn't find anything, so he was saying 'Don't get better too quick.' It upsets him now that he said that, in the light of what happened next. After the X-ray the consultant called us in and said there was a blockage. He showed us diagrams of the brain, but I couldn't take them in. It was all a blur after the word 'blockage'. He said she could have a tumour, cancer, meningitis – all these terrifying names. We didn't even know then that a tumour could be cancer.

While all the tests were going on Peter whipped out to get Joanne a Care Bear, because she'd been on at us for one for ages. In the next bed there was a little girl who'd knocked herself out in the playground at school, but the school hadn't been able to contact her parents yet. Joanne likes looking after people and she'd had the Care Bear for no time before she said, 'Let's give it to her. She's poorlier than I am and she's got no mam and dad with her. When they come she can give it back.'

Joanne was transferred by ambulance to Middlesbrough General Hospital – it's about seven or eight miles. By the time we got there it was 11 pm. Fortunately Sarah was staying the night with my friend Liz, whose child, Helen, is Sarah's best friend. So Sarah thought she was having a real treat!

11

BRAVE HEART

We stood on either side of Joanne while she had the scan, wearing heavy lead jackets for protection. Joanne's absolutely petrified of needles, and when they injected the dye she knew she mustn't move her head. I looked at her eyes and felt a terrible ache – tears were pouring from the corners down her cheeks. She was really brave and didn't move at all. But she was gripping my hand very tightly.

A bit later I heard someone say 'Tell the parents.' Then I knew it was bad news. The surgeon, Mr Nath, told us that there was a tumour and a cyst the size of a small egg. Can you imagine something so big in the brain of a young child? He said he would operate on the following Tuesday. She was so weak there was only a 60/40 chance of her coming through. Weeks or months later we would remember things that Mr Nath said, but when he was talking I didn't feel I was taking it in at all.

It was midnight. Joanne was given something to make her sleep and we were told to go home. I don't remember how we coped in those few days. It was like being dead while being alive. It was really Sarah that kept us going – having to keep up a front for her.

When Joanne was wheeled past us after the operation she was shaking all over. The nurse said it was because the brain had been tampered with and all her nerves had been upset. Mr Nath came out and said she was fine and we could see her in a few minutes when she had been wired up to the intensive care machines. I was so relieved I put my arms around him – I wanted to kiss him; and Peter was shaking his hand. Mr Nath was so embarrassed! He's a marvellous man and we owe everything to him.

Joanne came out just six days later, on our thirteenth wedding anniversary, and we opened a bottle of champagne. Our GP had gone to the hospital to visit her that day, and was astonished to be told that she'd been discharged. He called round and said, 'Can I go up and see her?' And

BRAVE HEART

I said, 'No, she's gone out for a walk with Peter.' Mr Nath wanted her to build up her strength quickly with lots of fresh air and exercise. When Joanne got back with Peter, our GP said he couldn't believe the transformation in her.

At the time of the operation Mr Nath told us that the tumour would recur, but that he and the pathologist disagreed about when. The pathologist said it was a quick-growing tumour, while Mr Nath didn't think it would come back until she was a teenager. Ten years ago they wouldn't even have been able to do the operation they did on Joanne. So we felt pretty confident that by the time she was a teenager more advances would have been made, and that the outlook was good if the tumour did come back. We had a smashing welcome home party in June, and made a video of it. It would have been easy to let everything prey on us, but we felt very lucky and just carried on with our lives.

But the pathologist was right. After ten or eleven months Joanne started getting headaches on and off again. At first I didn't panic about them. Then they started to get closer together. And then one day I remember we went out to the shops, and she stepped out of the car and was sick on the pavement. From then on she started being sick every time we went out in the car – and we knew. Afterwards Joanne said, 'I was frightened; I knew the tumour was coming back.' But she didn't tell us at the time.

The GP said there was no pressure on the brain, that it was impossible that it could have come back. But we knew. We phoned Mr Nath direct, and he told us to bring her straight in. They did the scan but we had to wait all day for Mr Nath to finish in the operating theatre so that he could look at the scan. At 9 pm the house doctor came in and told us to go home, because Mr Nath had been delayed. He said, 'Don't quote me, but I've looked at the scan and I think it's clear.'

BRAVE HEART

We went home and opened a bottle of wine – it was absolutely lovely. Then we spent the next three hours on the phone telling all the family. Peter has two brothers and sisters, and they've got children, so there's a lot of us when we get together! The moment he put the phone down, it rang. It was Mr Nath. I saw Peter's face fall. Mr Nath said he'd been trying to ring us all evening to tell us that the tumour was back.

Peter went to pieces. I'd never seen him like it, asking why it had to happen to our little girl. I used to be a Sunday School teacher, and we'd both been churchgoers in Sunderland, but when we moved to Stockton we'd drifted away. Anyway, we'd got to know the vicar when Joanne joined the Brownies, and so I rang him up. He was out at a meeting and his wife took the call. But although it was midnight he was there in five minutes. He stayed with us all night and helped us get through the worst.

When we went to the hospital the next day we could see the tumour immediately. Mr Nath said that this time it was virtually certain Joanne would be paralysed after the operation. Though I offered to cancel the holiday we had booked he told us to go because it would build her up, and it would almost certainly be the last holiday we'd ever have like it. Joanne had a wonderful time, dancing every night. We sat there watching her, with a terrible feeling welling up inside us.

Then Peter caught food poisoning and had to go to hospital. I was terrified that Joanne would catch the infection from him and the operation would have to be delayed. Finally he had to sign himself out, so that we could get back home. He lost two stone, and to start with wasn't allowed to go into Middlesbrough Hospital because of the risk of infection.

Before the operation Peter took us all to Scarborough as his birthday treat to us. The Royal Ballet was doing *Swan Lake*. It was a real killer. When the dying swan came on, Peter and I just sat there crying our eyes out. In

BRAVE HEART

a way I suppose it was a good thing, because it helped us to cry. The next morning was a horrible North-East morning, rainy and foggy, a kind of two more coats and a woolly hat job. Joanne just stood there on the front looking out to sea. We were shivering and damp and we couldn't get her to move – she was hypnotised. She said, 'Look, it's that ugly it's beautiful.' And she was right. We were so preoccupied we couldn't see it. But Joanne's like that, even when a thing's horrible she can still find something special in it.

Her second operation took seven hours. Mr Nath had told us it would be less. We watched nurses dashing in with bags of blood because Joanne lost a lot. Mr Nath said afterwards he couldn't believe how far the tumour had spread and that it had grown so quickly so soon. Miraculously she wasn't paralysed, but we were told that the prognosis wasn't good. Mr Nath said he couldn't give us any hope and that he couldn't operate again for at least two years whatever happened – May 1989 would be the earliest he could consider it. He gave Joanne six months to a year to live. Easter 1988 was the time limit – and Joanne's still alive today.

In May 1988, we said she could go anywhere in the world she wanted for a holiday, since she'd spent the last two Mays in hospital. She chose Disney World and so we blew our life savings on the trip. Some people said we shouldn't have, but you learn what's important to you.

Peter's in the hygiene and cleaning business. He started his own company cleaning hotel kitchens just after Sarah was born. Joanne's illness has had a devastating effect on the business. Peter wants to be with us all the time in case anything goes wrong. No employer would have let him have so much time off, and stop travelling. And now we travel all over the country for alternative therapies. So in that sense we've been fortunate in his job. But he's had to lay people off. When Joanne was first ill Peter fell behind with his VAT, and we let the tax and VAT people know. Then we had to write a letter giving the date of Joanne's appointments at the hospital, to prove it. I suppose people could make this up but it does seem a bit drastic. There were some evenings when we'd got the children to bed and we had a bit of free time and he could have settled down to the VAT I suppose, but after what were going through he would just have made mistakes. Anyway, as Peter says, he may not have the biggest cleaning company in the world, but who cares?

We've learnt not to hold grudges; we always put things right. I think of the King's Cross tragedy and those couples who left each other in the morning and then one of them died in the fire in the evening. In the beginning, because of the stress, we used to get at each other. But now I feel our problems have brought us closer together.

We've been careful, too, to make sure that Sarah knows she is loved just as much as Joanne. When we were invited to the Children of Courage Awards ceremony for Joanne to collect her award on December 14th, 1988, I insisted that Peter and Sarah came too. If Joanne is doing something with me, then Peter takes time with Sarah. One day Peter and I sat down and said to her, 'Do you think we love Joanne more than you? Because if you do we apologise.' And Sarah said she had been thinking that perhaps we did love Joanne more. There was a time when she started to get tummy aches and I even took her to the doctor. But in fact, though they did hurt, they were a way of getting attention. She knows now that she doesn't have to feel pain to get cuddles.

We've learned that you have to fight for your child when she's ill. A lot of people think we're barmy, but we've turned to alternative therapies, and showed Joanne how to visualise the cancer cells. Between the first and second operations we did nothing and the tumour grew back in ten months. Since the second operation we've cut out additives and preservatives as far as possible and eat as much organic produce as we can. We also make sure Joanne drinks only spring water and takes vitamins and minerals to try to help her immune system cope with the cancer. She's survived for longer than the gap between the two operations, and now she's already lived longer than even Mr Nath predicted.

Something like this changes your whole outlook on life. Now we live for each day, and we set goals to keep Joanne going. The next goal is the publication of this book. She wants to stay well to see it published, and we want to see it in every children's ward so that parents and children can learn from Joanne's experience and not be afraid.

K. Gillespie

Kathy Gillespie

BRAVE HEART

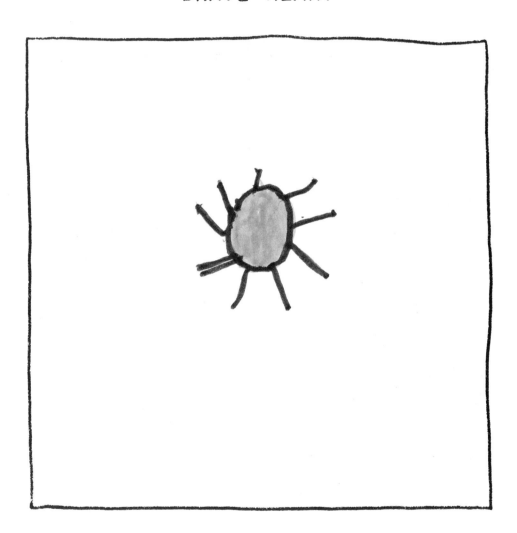

18

JOANNE'S DIARY

My name is Joanne Gillespie and I'm nine-and-a-half years old. I decided to write this book because when I was frightened and not sure of myself in hospital there was nothing for me to read. There were books for grown-ups but there were none for children. So, I decided to write this book for other children who are like me feeling frightened and ill. And I hope it will help them to feel a bit more sure of themselves.

It really all started with terrible headaches and sickness. The headaches started quite suddenly and they were very painful. At first, I thought my headaches were like everybody else's, but they just kept getting worse than any headache I had ever had before. It was awful. I had the sickness most of all when I got up and did something. Sometimes the headaches were so bad, I just stayed in bed and cried with the pain. My mam and dad got very

BRAVE HEART

worried. They took me to see our doctor who said it was just migraine because my mam and nana had it. And the doctor said it could have passed through the family. We went back home and the headaches didn't get better, they just got worse and worse.

My mam and dad got worried once more and took me to the doctor, yet again. This time when we were in the car my right side just went numb and I couldn't lift my right hand up to wave to a friend that I had seen. What was going on? I was frightened and didn't know what was happening. I couldn't lift my hand up! What could be the matter with me?

When we got to the doctor I couldn't walk in – my leg had done the same thing! What was the matter? What was happening? What was going on? I was very, very frightened and I didn't know what was happening. My dad had to carry me in. My mam and dad said to the doctor, 'This is not migraine.' The doctor replied, 'Well, I don't know what else it could be then.' He sent me down to North Tees Hospital to have some tests.

When I got into hospital, the nurses were really nice. They asked me loads of questions like how old I was, and gave me some medicine to try to stop me being sick that tasted like chalk – yuk – it didn't work though; I was sick all over the bed. I thought I would get into trouble but the nurses were really kind. They put a strap on my hand with my name on.

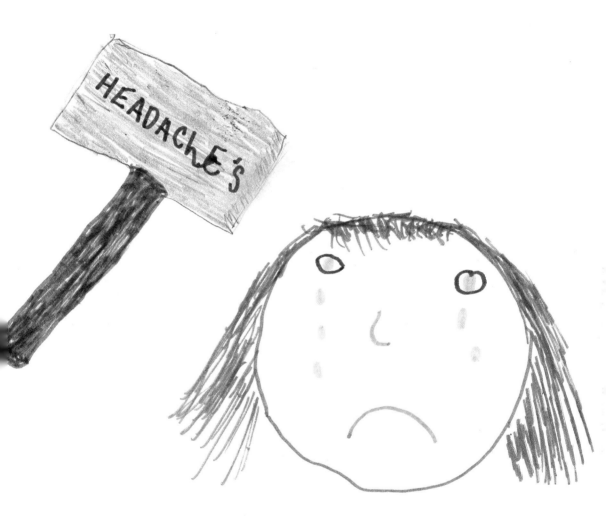

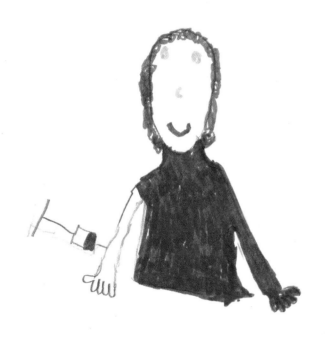

I felt as if there was no blood in really my right arm with all the needles

BRAVE HEART

Tests were carried out on me all day and I was seen by seven or eight doctors. The doctors were rougher than the nurses and they seemed to hurt more when they gave me the needles. I had quite a lot of blood tests and I knew that they would look at my blood with a microscope because I have one, but I thought that my blood was OK and didn't know what they were looking for or why they needed so much. My family and some of the nurses said that I should have no blood left in my right arm, but I knew I had plenty of blood left and I wished that they would take all they wanted in one go, share it out and then leave me alone. I also had my blood pressure taken and lots of X-rays. I'm glad all my family were there. It was really nice to know they all cared.

After the tests the doctors said that something was very wrong. They sent me down to Middlesbrough General Hospital to get a brain scan. My mam and dad told me I had to go to another hospital because the hospital I was in didn't have the right stuff to get me better.

I was sent to the Middlesbrough General in an ambulance with my mam and dad. When we got to Middlesbrough I had a scan. I didn't know what a brain scan was or how it worked. They told me that they needed pictures of the inside of my head and that was

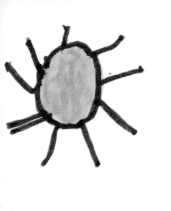
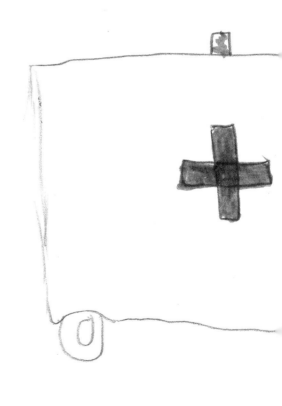

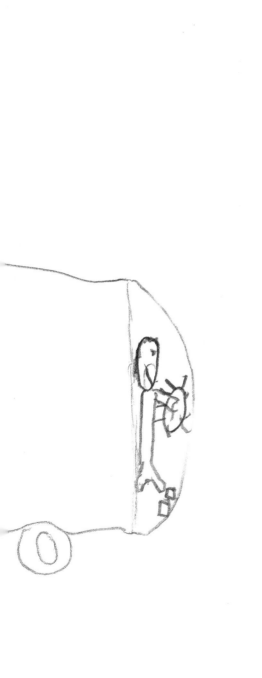

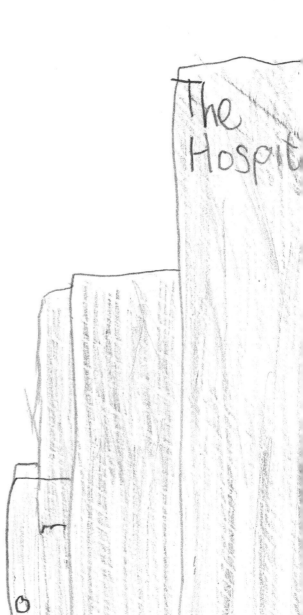

The Hospit

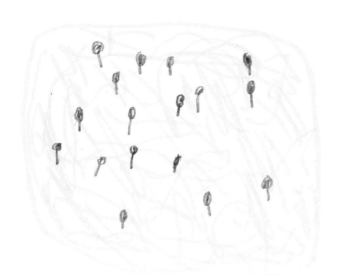

I felt like a pin cushion

BRAVE HEART

what a brain scan did. Guess what next? Yes – another needle! I was thinking I was going to be a *pin cushion* – needles here, needles there, needles nearly everywhere! Not only did I have to have another needle but I was also injected with some blue dye – yuk! It was horrible. It didn't hurt at all except for the needle but it had to be done, so I just let them get on with it. One of the doctors drew lines on my face so they could get the pictures in the right place. My mam and dad were still with me and they had to wear very special coats which were made of metal or something. I held their hands so it wasn't too bad, at least I wasn't on my own. The scan machine looked like a big washing machine that went round and round. I lay on a bed and my head went in the machine and it went round and round – not my head – just the machine!

After the scan there was some bad news for my mam and dad; I had a tumour and cyst. It would have to be operated on as soon as possible. The doctor who was going to operate on me was called Mr Nath. He is very nice. Mam and dad talked to him for ages and then told me what was wrong. They said a tumour was like a bruise that kept growing and a cyst was like a blister with water in it. They said that if I didn't let the doctor operate, my arm and leg would keep going funny and I would have to stop dancing. I know now that without the operation I would have died but mam and dad were too scared to tell me that then and didn't want to scare me.

BRAVE HEART

The doctors couldn't operate on me straightaway. I had to take steroids to stop the swelling in my head. It took about five days. On the day of my operation, Tuesday, May 13th, 1986, I wasn't allowed to eat or drink anything. By the time they took me to the operating theatre, I was starving. Mam and dad and my aunties were all joking about food. It made me a bit cross, but it stopped me from thinking about the operation. I wasn't frightened but I wasn't looking forward to it either.

When the nurses collected me from my room they told me that when I woke up I would be in a special ward where they would look after me. I got to the theatre; the doctors were wearing green coats, macs and rubber gloves. They worried me a bit. I knew they were going to get rid of the tumour and the cyst, which was good, but just seeing them made me scared, sort of like going to the dentist but worse. The nurse was going to give me an injection. She said it wouldn't hurt – fibber! – and that it had a special needle called 'Butterflies', then she gave me the injection. I felt very vague. I saw a man pulling his gloves on and then Mr Nath said, 'Come on Joanne.' I can't remember anything else after that until I woke up.

The operation lasted over four-and-a-half hours. When I woke up I had lots of wires attached to me and a drain and a bandage on my head. I was wrapped in a tin foil blanket and looked like a Christmas turkey ready to go into the oven. I had sticky things on

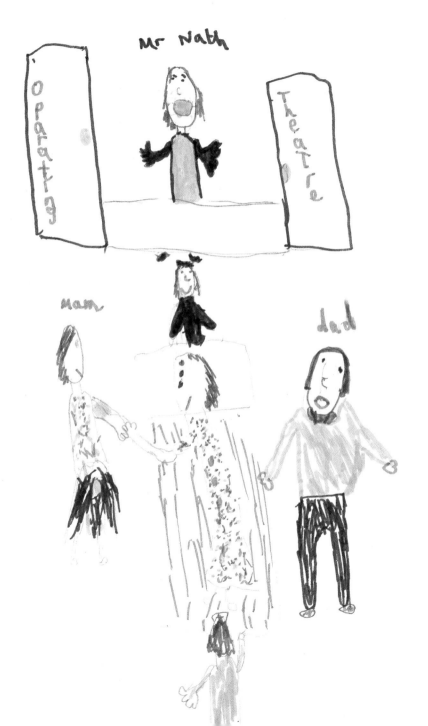

me and breathing machines next to me. My mam and dad said I was shivering and twitching. The first thing I can remember was feeling very, very hungry and I wanted to talk but I couldn't be bothered, so I just looked at things and made signs. My lips were very dry and I wanted a drink too. Later the nurses came to see me and asked me questions: 'What was my name?' 'How old was I?' 'Did I know where I was?' I told them I was in Ward 18. They were impressed. I know now that they were checking my memory and speech. Then they started to tickle my feet and asked me if I could feel it. I thought the nurse was being silly, of course I could feel it, it was my head that had the operation, not my feet. They were trying to make sure I could still feel them, but I was tired and it seemed a stupid thing to do at the time.

I stayed in Intensive Care till I could go back to the Children's Ward. I had my own little room – posh eh? All my family were waiting to see me, aunties, uncles, nana, everybody – I must have been really popular! They were not popular with the nurses and got thrown out because there were too many in the room. Still, it felt very nice to be loved so much.

For the next few days the nurses came in about every hour or so to take my temperature and blood pressure and look into my eyes. I asked if I could take the nurse's blood pressure as they had taken mine so often and she said I could. So I did but I didn't know

BRAVE HEART

what it meant. I knew how to do it because mine was taken all the time and I watched, but I needed some help and didn't understand a word when she tried to explain how it worked.

I had sort of clips in my head and they were taken out on May 16th. The clips are like staples – they're used instead of stitches and helped my head grow back together again. Some of them hurt because they had been put in tightly. When the nurse started to take them out it didn't feel very nice and she said she would only take a few out that day and come back the next day to take out the rest. Because I felt I wanted to get it over and done with I told her to take them out all at once. So she did. Just remember to try and relax and not cry, and it soon passes. I kept a tight hold of my mam's hand and that helped too. I was so brave, I got a Bravery Award – *Five Star* – I'm very proud of it.

The nurses were very nice. We liked telling each other jokes, although I drove them mad with my joke book. They tried really hard to make me happy – they were really good. Sometimes they said I was a pest when I asked them lots of questions about their boyfriends and tried to get my Aunty Joan a doctor for a boyfriend, because she said he was dishy – when I told the doctor I think she was very embarrassed!

When my bandage came off, my hair was all sticky and horrible. I had a big bald patch where my head had been shaved for the operation. The nurse spread some stuff onto my head so no water could get into it. Then she washed and dried my hair with a blower. I was a bit nervous but she was very gentle. Having my hair done felt really nice.

I wanted to get up as soon as possible and as there were lots of little babies in the hospital I was able to help the nurses with them. I love babies. I had no pain but Mr Nath told us to be careful and not bump my head. That would stop me from riding my bike. I could eat normally but sometimes the meals were awful. My mam and dad would bring me something to eat.

One day the vicar from our church, David Jones, came to see me. I was always trying to keep myself cheerful in hospital and I said to him 'Did you come in a rush?' The vicar said, 'No, Why?' and I said, 'Because you've got your shirt on back to front!' We all had a good laugh at that. Then, after he had gone, my mam and dad said they had felt like sliding under the bed.

Anyway, my cheekiness caught up with me one day because the hospital teacher said that as I was feeling so well, I could try to do some school work – I felt really fed up!

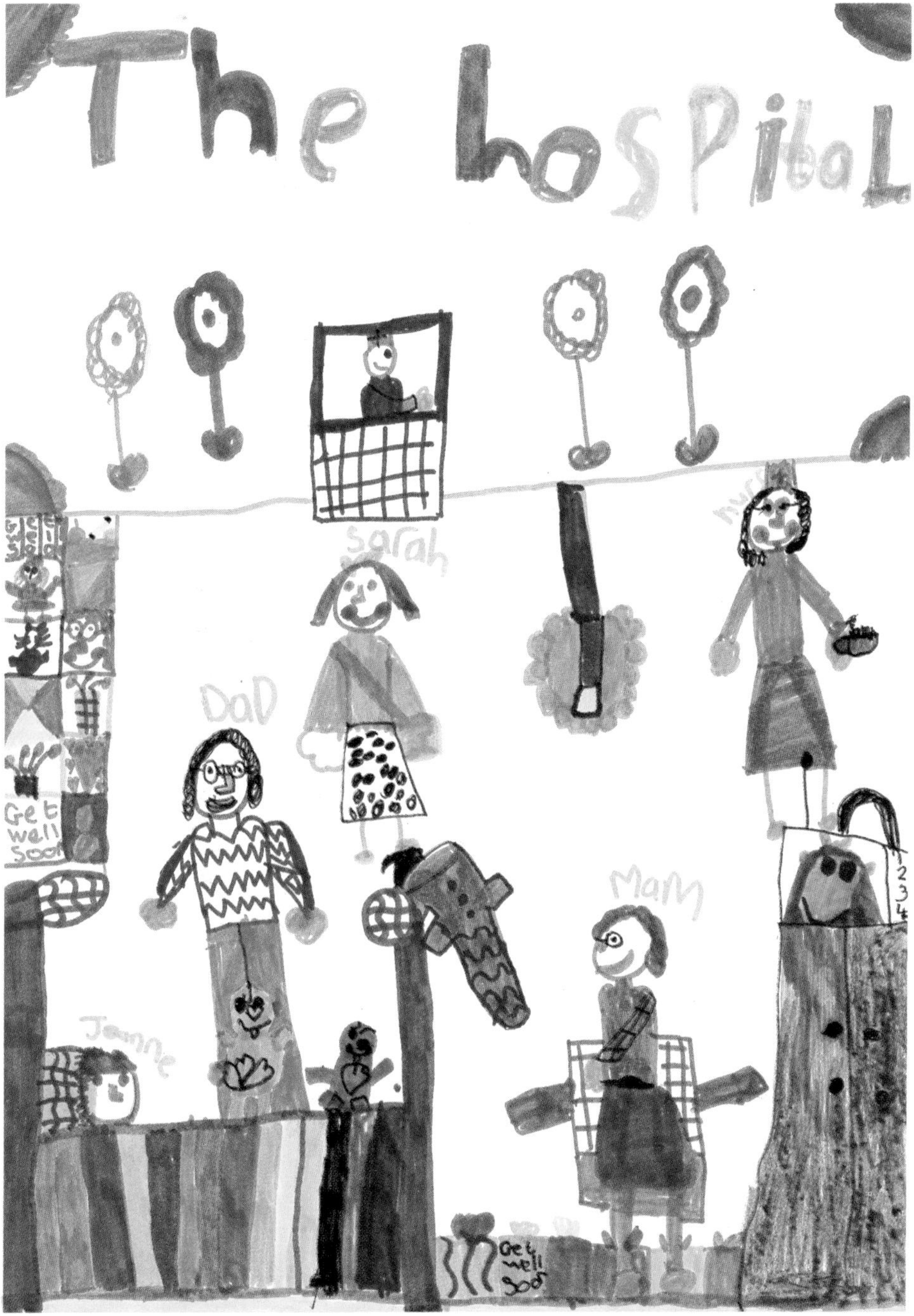
The hospitaL
sarah
DaD
MaM

BRAVE HEART

I came home on May 19th. I must have been the happiest person alive. It was my mam and dad's thirteenth wedding anniversary. It certainly wasn't unlucky for them. My mam said it was the best anniversary present they had ever had. We even opened a bottle of champagne to celebrate. But I didn't get drunk!

My doctor came to see me and he thought I'd be upstairs in bed, but I'd gone for a walk with my dad. He was surprised that I was normal and walking about.

I've still got the lovely pictures that my six-year-old sister, Sarah, drew me when I was in hospital and two of them are used in this book on pages 8 and 33. She really cheered me up. She told me jokes and brought me cards from school and came to visit me all the time. She told me what was happening at dancing. A lot of people got their own back on me when I was in hospital, telling me jokes instead of me telling them. But I'm really glad my sister took it so well. She knew I was poorly but I don't think she knew how poorly. I didn't know that so I don't suppose Sarah would have known. I think she must have been a bit frightened for me. She was only five then. I'm just glad that she understood. I think I am very lucky to have such a special sister and although we fight sometimes I love her very much and it was nice to sleep in our own room again.

Everything was all right. We had a big Welcome Home Party in our garden. All our family and friends were invited – we had a barbecue with lots of games like knobbly knees, three-legged races, pass the parcel, and lots more. My mam made a special cake and my dad put icing on it saying 'Welcome Home Joanne'. It was a lovely day.

I didn't go back to school straightaway. I was off for a couple of months but, surprisingly, when I did get back to school, I really enjoyed it – well, for a couple of months anyway! I started going to dancing again at about the same time as I went back to school. I didn't feel tired, or anything like that, but there was just a slight twitch in my right hand which I still get now. What happens really is my fingers curl up and I can't push them back again. I have to use up all my strength to push the fingers out again. It hurts a lot but I don't moan. If things like that happen, you can't moan or it won't get better. You've got to fight it and that's exactly what I'm doing, and it seems to be getting better. I was given some medicine and tablets to take – steroids and epilim to stop me having fits.

My mam and dad didn't tell me what the doctor had said about the dangers of having the operation, that there was a chance that I might die because I was so weak – they didn't want me to be frightened. After I came home, I was feeling really fed up one day. Why me? Why did I have to be poorly? I thought I was the unluckiest person alive. Mam and dad sat me down and told me

BRAVE HEART

just how lucky I was. I could have lost my speech or been paralysed. I could have died. Without the operation I would have. It was a big shock. Me in a wheelchair? Not being able to tell jokes or play games or dance? We all cried a bit but I knew I wasn't as unlucky as I thought.

Everything was fine for about ten or eleven months. And then disaster struck. I started getting headaches and sickness again. I was a bit frightened but I didn't realise the tumour was coming back until the headaches got really bad again. My mam and dad took me back to the doctor. The doctor looked into my eyes and said it wasn't the tumour coming back and there was nothing to worry about. But my mam and dad knew the symptoms. So, when we got back, they phoned Mr Nath, the surgeon, at the hospital. He said I had to go straight there for another brain scan. My mam and dad thought it was the cyst filling up again. But after the scan Mr Nath took my mam and dad into his office and told them that the tumour had grown back again. It had grown over where the cyst had been last year. He said he would have to operate on me again.

We had a holiday in Menorca booked and my mam said that she would cancel the holiday so that Mr Nath could do the operation

THE

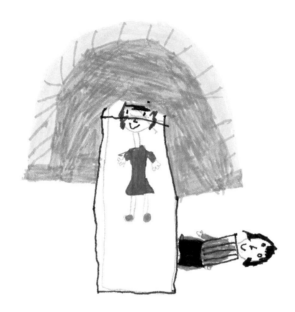

SCAN

GOOD

LUCK

BEAR

BRAVE HEART

straightaway. Mr Nath asked me whether I wanted the operation before or after the holiday – I found out later that he'd asked because he thought that after the operation I wouldn't be able to dance and I'd be in a wheelchair, and might lose my voice. When mam and dad told me what Mr Nath had said, I couldn't really believe it. The only thing I did understand was that I had to have the operation or else I wouldn't be able to dance. Nothing was going to stop me from dancing and that was really all that mattered to me. I wasn't told then that I could die – mam and dad only told me after the operation. Mr Nath told mam that we should all enjoy a good holiday and he would do the operation when we came back.

When we went on holiday I wasn't worried about the operation. I was doing all the things I wanted to do and just had a good time. I didn't know what might happen in the future and didn't realise how much my parents must have been worrying. Now, I wish I could have helped them and told them not to worry but, at the time, I didn't think there was anything to worry about except that I was to have an operation. While we were on holiday I won a dancing medal, because I was the best dancer. I felt very good and happy when I was presented with the medal. I know my mam and dad and sister were proud too.

I had my operation on May 7th, 1987. It lasted for seven hours.

THE
NEEDLE!

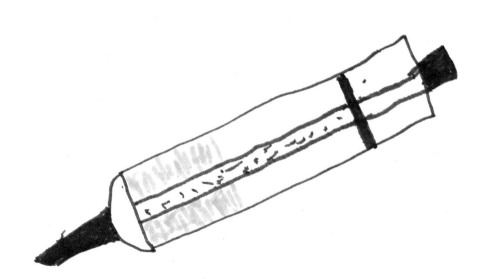

BRAVE HEART

My mam and dad and sister and my whole family were very, very worried, and I was very scared as they wheeled me into the operating theatre. The nurses and doctors remembered me. They were glad to see me – well, not glad to see me but glad to see me – if you know what I mean. This time they gave me a special sort of cream on the top of my head and on top of both of my hands. When I went into the theatre, and I had the needle, I didn't feel a thing. Isn't that good? Also, they only did a couple of routine tests which is not bad, if you're afraid of needles like I am.

When I went into the operating theatre I brought with me one of my Care Bears which I had received last year as a present when I was in hospital. I brought 'Good Luck Bear' which my mam and dad had given to me. When I woke up from the operation 'Good Luck Bear' had a bandage on his head like me and he was attached to a lemonade drip – made out of paper and string. That helped to cheer me up a bit, especially as when I came out of the theatre, I had this funny needle stuck into me. It hurt so much I was screaming and clutching my mam's arm. The needle was being pushed in, then a little bit further, and a little bit further. I think they were giving me this injection because I couldn't lift my right hand. It was stiff again, and so was my right leg, too. I thought the doctor was being unkind, though, because my right arm was stiff and I couldn't feel anything yet he had to go and put the needle in my *left* arm where I could feel all the pain. Why couldn't he just put the needle in my *right* arm and then I wouldn't have felt anything? Oh well – I suppose the doctor had his reasons.

I was back in Intensive Care again and once more I had wires attached to me and a heart machine that made a funny noise. This time when the nurse tickled my feet I could not feel anything on my right foot. My right hand was just the same and my mam and dad thought that I was going to be paralysed just like the doctor had said. For a while I was worried but Mr Nath came in and said it was natural after an operation like mine. I could still talk though and did quite a lot! When I was sent back to the Children's Ward I could still not feel anything in my leg, but I was cheered up a lot when I saw all my Care Bears with bandages and oxygen masks on. My dad called them the 'Intensive Care Bears' and we took some photographs of them which I still have.

While I was feeling strange I had to use the bedpan which was horrible – I hated it. Every time I went on it I wet the bed. I was determined to go to the proper toilet. I couldn't walk properly, so I had to just put up with it for a little while, but as soon as my leg began to get a little stronger I was determined to use the toilet. I leaned on my mam and made myself walk to the toilet and every day I got stronger – I didn't get in a wheelchair because I fought it.

BRAVE HEART

My mam was determined to help me as well, and she didn't mind – and I was glad. The nurses didn't want me to as they said I wasn't even allowed out of bed and I had a bit of an argument with them because I insisted and refused to use a bedpan. Day after day my right arm and leg recovered more feeling. Soon I could walk to the toilet just holding my mam's hand. It was a great feeling!

Again I had to have clips or staples in my head and I had them taken out on May 12th. Some of them came out easily and I got another Bravery Award after they'd taken them out. The nurses said I was so brave that I deserved it. The nurses had tried their best to cheer me up saying, 'It'll be over soon, Joanne.' I know they were fibbing but they were trying to make me feel better.

I got lots of visitors in hospital and one of them was my Headmistress, Mrs Carnell, and my teacher, Miss Hutchinson. Mrs Carnell brought me a joke book as a present because she knew I liked telling jokes. I have lots of joke books and the one Mrs Carnell brought me I had already got and I told her so. (My mam and dad said afterwards that they felt like slipping under the bed again!) But Mrs Carnell didn't mind and said that after I had returned to school she would arrange a date to take me to the bookshop and choose a different book. I was glad and had something to look forward to.

BRAVE HEART

While I was in hospital I had to do lots of exercises to help to strengthen my hand and arm. Some of these were boring, so my mam and I decided to practise together to music. One of my favourites was anything by 'Bucks Fizz' – their music is really lively and we made up lots of good moves. It helped to make all the boring exercises more interesting.

I found it really hard to write and I was given a special holder for my pen to try and help me. I also got a special knife and fork with thick handles so I could grip them easily. I've still got them because sometimes it's difficult to hold a normal fork, but I'm getting used to it and am better with it now. I had jig-saws to do, too, all to help my hand to get stronger. I started writing with my left hand when I went back to school because I felt silly that my writing looked so bad. People said, 'Well, you've had an operation; just do the best you can.' But I wanted it to be better. So I started writing with my left hand and found that I could write better with it than I could with my right hand. I think if you really try hard to do something you can if you are really determined.

After the operation the doctor said I would need a course of radiotherapy treatment to try and kill off any cancer cells that might have been left over from the operation. When I started my treatment, I didn't know what it was or how it would work. Just a big word. It kind of scared me.

exercises for Arm

My MaM

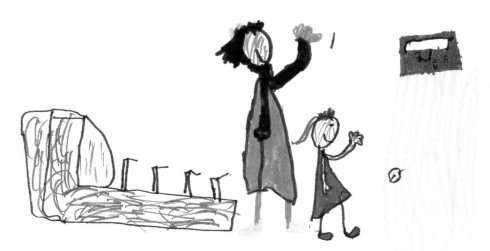

BRAVE HEART

The worst bit was getting my mask made. I needed the mask to stop me moving my head when I was having the radiotherapy treatment. You have to keep completely still so the machine can take pictures of the cancer in your body and fight the bad cells. If you move it may kill the good white cells too. To make the mask my hair was covered with a sort of swimming cap and then they put yukky grease stuff on my face and covers on my eyes, mouth and ears. I was told not to talk for about ten minutes (which is not very easy for me!) and I had to lie very still, because if I moved my head or face at all we would have to start again. They patted plaster of Paris on my face only leaving two breathing holes for my nose. They put more and more on my face. I couldn't see or talk. It was dark and scarry and I didn't know where I was. Mam held my hand and dad my side but I still felt all alone. When the plaster of Paris dried it was lifted off my face and I could sit up – I was really glad. I hadn't moved so the first mask was OK. The plaster mask was used to make a copy of my head. When I finished my radiotherapy treatment they gave me it to keep. I keep my hat and sunglasses on it now.

My mask fitted well and I started my treatment on May 19th – mam and dad's wedding anniversary again. After having the mask done I was a bit scared but it was easy. You just lie there and lights come out of the machine and they move it about. That's all. I just

BRAVE HEART

listened to some of my favourite music tapes while mam and dad could see me on a little television. After a couple of minutes (well, it seemed like that to me anyway), it was finished and I didn't know what I'd been worrying about. Silly me, because cancer cells like people to worry. I know I do worry sometimes, but don't worry too much if you don't want the cancer cells to win.

I had about twenty sessions and every time I came I would help the ladies to make tea and cheer people up who looked so down and miserable. Their faces nearly touched the floor. There were some children who looked really sad and down, but what surprised me was that it was mostly the parents who looked down and said 'Oh dear, what am I going to do, I'm going to be sick.' Some people even went in with sick bowls at the ready. Well, I don't think that's being very positive; I think it's being silly. I couldn't believe it. I believe that if people trust in themselves and God and say 'I'm going to make it; I'm going to do it', they *are* going to do it. I know that some people are saying, 'Oh dear, this is never going to work, why am I taking all these tablets? I'm getting fed up with all this. Why did God choose me?' I believe that God didn't choose anybody. It just happens to people. I feel that if they want to get better, they can get better, but they need to try. Some people don't seem as if they want to fight, but they must, otherwise they must like being poorly. I have only got one life and I am going to live it as long as

BRAVE HEART

I am here! *I am going to fight. And I am going to win*! What helped me through this is wanting to be a dancer so much that I have fought and fought my illness, yet I was supposed to be dead at Easter and I am still here. So I believe that if you face it and you believe, you will get better. For instance, I was never sick when I was having radiotherapy. Everybody else was and they were the ones that went around feeling sorry for themselves, wishing that they were dead. I was all right because I believe in *me* and that's the most important thing – to believe in yourself.

My last visit for radiotherapy was on June 17th. I was given steroid tablets because of the operation to stop the swelling and pressure. They made me very fat but fortunately they didn't make me feel sick. In fact, I take so many vitamins now that people call me 'The Professional Pill Popper'.

Radiotherapy also makes your hair fall out – well my hair didn't exactly fall out; it was just that if I pulled, hair just came out in my hand. Sometimes it fell out on my pillow when I was asleep and itched me so badly that it woke me up in the night. So I decided one morning that I would pull it all out and the final score was a little bit in the front and a little bit at the back. That was when my dad started calling me Baldilocks. I didn't feel anything about going bald – I just felt it was me with not a lot of hair on top of my head. Some people stare – mostly grown-ups and it isn't nice. I started to wear a badge saying 'It's rude to stare'. Some of my friends still played with me, but others stayed away. I tried to please them by wearing a wig, but that didn't please them either, 'Joanne's got a wig on, Joanne's got a wig on' they'd cry. In the end I just ignored them. If you've got a problem like that, ignore them and they'll just get used to it in the end.

When I went back to school, I felt angry but I found out then who were my real friends and, surprisingly, I had a lot of really good friends who didn't care whether I had hair or not. My sister was helping me all the time and, when people wouldn't play with me at first, she would. Sometimes, I couldn't play with my friends because I couldn't run very fast at the time, so I would play with my friend Nicola. But I'm very glad Sarah was there. Sometimes, when I play with Sarah, it's better than playing with my friends.

I am grateful to Mr Nath – he is brilliant – and to all the doctors and nurses who looked after me. I am going to do everything I can to stop the tumour from coming back. The hospital has helped me a lot, but now it's up to me. My mam and dad told me when I got back from the hospital – before I even started school – everything that was wrong with me and what would have happened to me if I hadn't had the operation, and now I think I understand what cancer is. Mr Nath still hadn't said to me that it was cancer. One day I went to see Mr Nath and said to him 'You can give me a scan,

White good cells

me

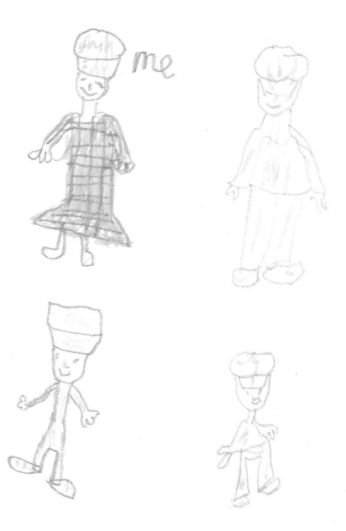

grey
bad
cells

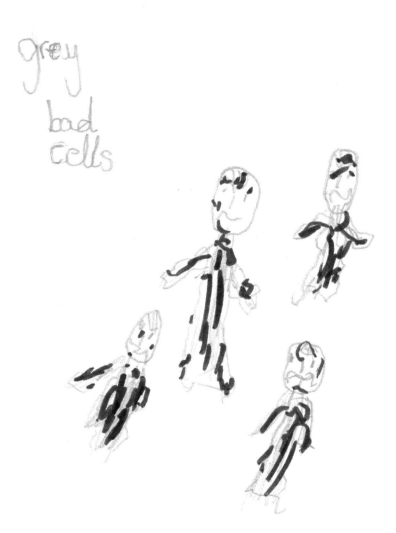

BRAVE HEART

I haven't got the cancer,' but he said, 'Well, you didn't have cancer anyway, you only had a tumour.' After that, I didn't quite know what he was talking about but my mam and dad said, when we got in the car, that he said that because he didn't want me to get frightened. We tell each other jokes each time when I go to see him. Most grown-ups are afraid of cancer themselves and think that children will be even more frightened, so they don't tell them everything. I'm glad that my mam and dad talked to me and explained as much as they could – I'm glad they were honest.

While I was in hospital the second time my mam and dad read lots of books about alternative medicine so that we could try and help ourselves.

I started to see Matthew Manning, a healer, in May. He taught me how to visualise. You can visualise anything. I visualise cancer cells as grey weak soldiers and my good cells as a strong white army with good fighters. I make the two armies fight and see all the grey soldiers smashed up and killed – no prisoners my mam and dad say – and I always make sure of that. Then a big waterfall runs right through my body washing away all the dead soldiers. I do this listening to music, sometimes soft music with no words. Then I visualise myself as I want to be – strong, healthy and *dancing*.

BRAVE HEART

I want to be a dancer and I am going to be a dancer – cancer won't stop me!

During my radiotherapy I did lots of visualising and I still do it now. I imagined nice things like picnics, holidays and dancing, things that cancer wants to stop, but I'm not letting it. All through my radiotherapy I had no sickness at all and I believe that visualising helps because I'll tell you a story about when I was having my radiotherapy. When you are having radiotherapy, it kills a lot of bad cells but it also kills some of your good white cells. Well, my white cell count was too low, so if my white cells didn't increase, I would have to stop radiotherapy. So I went home and visualised our liquidiser and I imagined I was putting into it all the good food – carrots, fruit, nuts, muesli, currants – things that are good for you. Then I visualised, instead of them coming out as chopped carrots, fruit and things like that, I imagined that they came out as white good cells. I did this with lots and lots of things and, by the time I'd finished, I had got thousands and thousands of white cells that I had imagined. The next day, when we went to the radiotherapy, the blood count was raised and I was able to go on with the radiotherapy again. I believe now that it must work because my white cell count went straight up and I think that was because of the visualisation. And that's why I always use visualisation. Some people say visualisation doesn't work but I

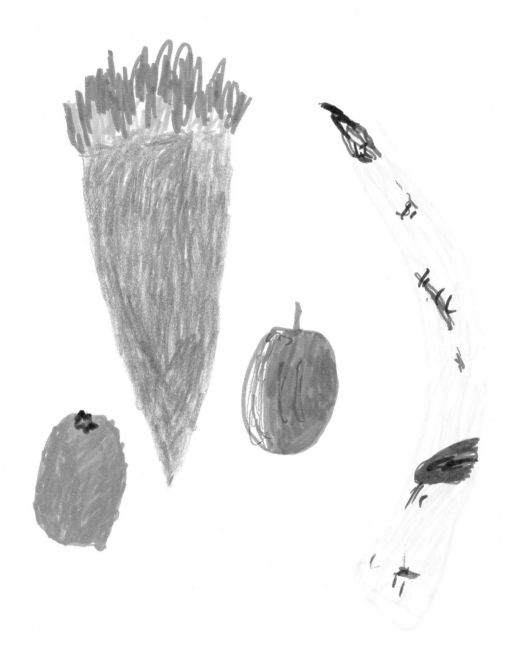

BRAVE HEART

believe that it helps you. If anybody asks me what they could do because their counts are low or something, I would tell them to visualise.

When I was home again I was taking about eight steroid tablets a day and I had to get off them. When I got down to two tablets one day, after school, I was sitting down and, all of a sudden, I started talking funnily. I tried to tell my mam and dad but all that came out was 'blurp, blurp, blurp', or something like that. I was shaking and my voice was funny and I wondered what was happening. My dad took me back to hospital at a belt of a million miles an hour I should say. At the hospital I was given – yes – you've guessed it, *another needle*! I had very bad headaches and was crying with them all the time. I was wondering why it had suddenly happened; I was feeling fine before it started. I was shivering and shaking and I felt really, really frightened. What was happening to me? I couldn't even stop myself. My voice had just gone funny. What's happened? I thought to myself. It got worse and worse and I had a fit. My mam and dad and Sarah were terrified but they told me Sarah was very good. She helped to hold me and wiped my mouth when it dribbled. She drew me a picture of Brave Heart Lion. I still have it, you can see it on page 8 of this book. My mam put a cold cloth on my head to try to ease the pain.

It had been a stroke and it made my right arm and leg go all weak again. I think I stayed in hospital for one night and they kept checking me to see if I was all right. When I could go home my head felt a lot better. The doctors, nurses and my mam and dad told me that I'd had a fit and I had to do all the exercises over again to get my arm and leg stronger. I got a bit cross about doing them again but I was going to keep doing them until it stopped happening. What I did was, when I got home, I either did them when people were around or I went into my bedroom to do them. I've got another physiotherapist who comes to my house sometimes – her name is Mrs Johnson. Some of the exercises she gives me are absolutely boring, but I can see that I am getting stronger each day. My leg and my arm still go funny sometimes, mostly my arm, but I *will* beat it and I hope I don't visit the hospital in a long long time.

Another of the alternative therapies my mam and dad found out about was the Bristol Cancer Diet and natural healing. The Bristol Cancer Diet is 75 per cent raw food and fresh vegetables. No tea, coffee or dairy products. I think that the Bristol diet helps a lot. I've not been in hospital since I've been on this diet and I think it is the diet which is keeping me out. It does not worry me that children have chocolate bars, sweets and things like that, because I know that they've got colours in and anway I've never had a filling since I've been out of hospital. I've had an old filling put in again but I haven't had a new one and I think that's because I don't have any sugar, sweets or anything. People think I miss chocolates and ice-cream but I don't. I can have carob which hardly has any sugar in it and soya ice-cream. So I'm not really bothered what other children eat, but sometimes I do have a treat like a Mars bar or a packet of crisps.

There are lots of other things I can change, but we have to look for them. I only drink bottled water and herb teas. You soon get used to them. I eat lots of mung beans and things, and drink carrot juice and whenever possible mam tries to get me only organic food, that means that it hasn't been sprayed with chemicals. That's what the Bristol diet is all about – no chemicals or colours or anything like that. My mam, dad and sister follow the same diet too, but they are not as strict as me.

Because I don't have all the foods that most people have I also have to take lots of vitamins and minerals. My Naturopath doctor, Mr Howarth, helps me with them. I take vitamins A, B, C and E, organic Germanium tablets, evening primrose, zinc and selenium and royal jelly and lots, lots more. Some people think I should rattle when I walk – my mam and dad understand what they are for but I just take them – it's much better than having needles!

Mam and dad also take me to a Support Group where there are other people with cancer. We all help each other and have a good talk. I also go to the Children's Cancer Help Centre in Kent, where we meet other children and draw pictures of what we think our disease looks like. I met a boy with leukaemia and had a long talk with him. Mums and dads get help too.

Laughing helps to keep you well too, that's why I tell lots of jokes. We all laugh in our house – my dad is really mad! We have lots of fun and do everything together – none of us are scared of cancer, we all stick together.

Some people think I don't know that cancer can kill you, but I do. Cancer will never kill me though – if I die it will be because God wants me.

You have got to face the fact that you have got a tumour or cancer, but it's not just you who has it – there are thousands of other people like us who have got it. Please don't give up – *there is a way*, but it is different for everybody. This has been my way, it might not be any good for you, it might not work for me, but every day is special so you must find your way and fight it. You are not a prisoner!

Sometimes I worry about my mam and dad even though they tell me not to. In case I didn't win my fight I told my mam and dad that whatever happens I will always be with them if they close their eyes and look for me. Once I had said that and got it out of the way I could carry on with my fight.

Crying. Crying is all right and you have got to do it sometimes.

BRAVE HEART

If you feel as if you have got to cry, please do, but don't do it all the time. There is one thing to remember above all, you have only one life so try to make the most of it. I'd just like to say don't give in, there is a lot to life, there is a lot worth living for in it. I know that because I'm going to be a dancer. Maybe you know what you'd like to be when you grow up. Maybe a nurse or a typer, maybe even a dancer like me. But don't give in though. Trust in yourself and God, and you'll be all right. God is on *your* side, He will help you.

I have lots more to say, but I can't find the right words to say them with, just try to understand what I have been telling you.

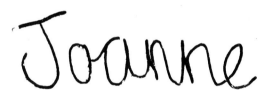

BRAVE HEART

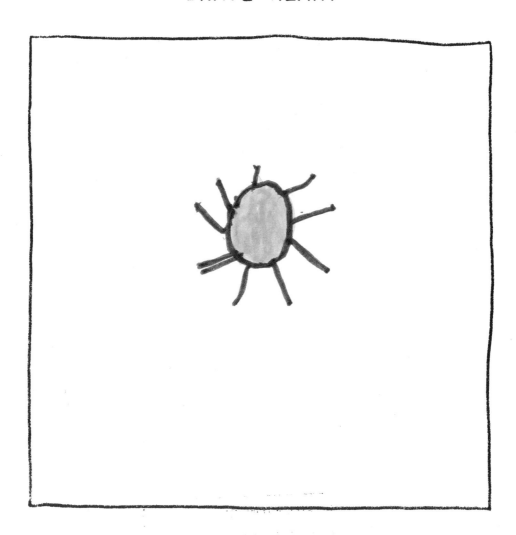

BRAVE HEART

1988

~~I wish~~

I wish that all the wars would end
That every person could be a friend
I wish that the world starving had more
to eat.
I wish I could buy the field down
our street
I'd Build a house have a treat with saugages
Beef Burgers cream cakes and sweets
invite all the people Ive wanted to
meet like people off fame or wayne
sleep
I wish I had a cruser and a caravan
I wish I was famous
I wish everyone was as happy as I
am.